Herbal Medicine

The Powerful Uses of Herbal Remedies for Natural Healing, Longevity and Health

Robert S. Lee

Contents

Chapter 1. What Dried Herbs Are & How to Dry Them

When you're using dried herbs, you can always buy them. However, they won't have the same potency as if you harvested and dried them yourself. When you dry your own herbs, you know exactly how old they are. You should never keep dried herbs and expect a high potency after six to eight months. Though, if you're cooking with them or looking for a mild effect, then it's okay to keep dried herbs for up to a year before throwing them out. When you dry your own herbs, make sure that you properly label everything, as many herbs will look the same after they're dried.

Air Drying:

After you cut and rinse the herbs, you are going to want to dry them. Most herbs will need to be air-dried. The next step is removing the leaves from the lower stems. Turn the branches upside down, and then you'll want to remove the leaves until you hit the upper stem. The buds and growing tips should be left alone because they are the most pungent.

Next, once you have properly prepared the stems make sure to tie some together. It is best to not tie more than six or seven together. If the herb is high in moisture then you can use smaller bunches so that it doesn't mildew while you try and make sure that it dries.

The tied branches are then going to need put in a paper bag. Make sure to gather the bag at the end where the stems are tied. The bag will need many holes or tears put into it, as ventilation is required. The bag should not be filled tightly, and a lot of room will be necessary. The name and date on each bag. When they're dried, they'll all look similar.

You can also spread the branches over a dehumidifier if you want to. Just make sure to spread them up loosely, allowing the air to circulate around them. This will help to dry them out faster. If you have a high quantity of herbs, this may take too long.

If you are still sticking with air drying, you are going to need to hang the bag up. The room should be airy and warm. A lot of people prefer to hang them in an attic because it's a room that usually works perfectly. You'll need to leave them alone to dry. Always check for signs of mold growth, but they'll need to dry for two weeks. If you find mold, you'll need to toss the entire batch.

Once they're dry, you'll have to separate the leaves away from the stems. The stems are going to need to be discarded. You can then crush the leaves. Whole herbs are usually better, and you can always crush them later. If they're not crushed, they'll have a more potent flavor.

A Little About Storing:

After you dry the herbs, you're going to need to store them. Always make sure to keep herbs out of the light, as it's best to help them keep their potency. Glass, airtight containers are best. Of course, you can also use zip locked bags as well, putting them in the plastic or glass container afterwards. Some people will even use vacuum sealed bags too, as it'll remove all of the air. It'll help your herbs to last a little longer.

Using the Oven Method for Drying:

You don't have to wait two weeks if you don't want to. You can actually dry herbs with your oven as well, and this is a very popular drying method. Some herbs you have to actually use this type of method for because otherwise they will mold. There are some herbs that have a high moisture content, which you'll be able to tell almost immediately. Lemon balm and mints are examples of this.

When using the oven drying method, you'll need to keep the oven on from 140 to 200 degrees, as anything higher will result in much more tasteless herbs. They'll also lose potency when it comes to using them in herbal remedies. You will not put the herbs in the oven when it's at this temperature. Let it run for about twenty minutes, and afterwards you're going to want to turn the oven off. Next, pop in the herbs and leave them there until they dry out.

Keep herbs separate, usually it's best to use separate trays, as it will result in you being able to tell which herbs are which after drying. It can be dangerous if you are using the wrong dried herb in your recipe, so proper labeling is best.

Using a Food Dehydrator for Drying:

If you have a food dehydrator, you can use it to dry your herbs as well, and once again this is a very popular method because it is easier and less time consuming. All you have to do is spread the herbs out on the food dehydrator's rack. Make sure that there aren't any clumps. It's best to use a food dehydrator if you're

6

trying to dry a large amount of herbs, especially those that are high in moisture content.

It makes everything a little easier, and you won't have to wait as long to get your herbs ready for use. Some people will just buy their dried herbs, but having your own will help make sure you have a higher potency and flavor in your herbs, which you wouldn't get from store bought herbs.

Chapter 2. Dried Herbs & Their Uses in Teas

When you're using dried herbs, the best and most common way to use them is in a tea. This is because you can rehydrate them in a way, allowing them to release a lot of their helpful properties, and it'll help you to feel a little better. Often, a tea will help you in ways that other dried herb uses just can't, and they're easy to make.

Keep in mind that when you're using an herbal tea, it is best to stay away from sugar. Sugar can aggravate a variety of ailments, and it is best to stick with honey. Honey has many antioxidants and is much less likely to harm you while you're trying to healing yourself. It is a natural way that you can sweeten your herbal tea. Lemon can also be added to almost any herbal tea, as it's up to preference.

Tea #1 A Tea for Sleep

You'll find that this tea is a powerful way to help you sleep, and it'll help you to get better rest as well. Some people report that they do not dream when using this tea, but many others will find that there is no difference than if they fell asleep naturally, and dreams do persist past it. None of these herbs need to be fresh, and dried herbs will do just fine.

Ingredients:

1. 1 Teaspoon Passionflower
2. ½ Teaspoon Mint
3. ½ Teaspoon Lemon Balm

The Reasons Behind It:

9

You'll find that both passionflower and lemon balm is known for its sedative properties. A strength of a tea will usually depend on the herbal amount as well as how long you steep it. The mint is known to help release tension as well, helping you to release yourself from anxiety and stress. It will also help you to relieve stomach upset, allowing you to get to sleep a little easier.

Tea #2 A Tea for Arthritis

Arthritis is a pain that you shouldn't have to deal with, and dried herbs can help you with arthritis when taken internally as well. Just make sure that you take it at least once daily if you want an effect. It should steep for about five minutes before you add honey or lemon.

Ingredients:

1. 1 Teaspoon Dried Ginger

2. ½ Teaspoon Turmeric

3. 1 Teaspoon Rosemary

The Reason Behind It:

Ginger is known to help with inflammation, as well as Turmeric. Rosemary is also an herb that you can easily grow in your garden, and it's great to add to the mix as well due to its anti-inflammatory properties. You will often find these ingredients in your spice cabinet, and they're already dried. This makes it extremely easy to make this tea and take it for arthritis. You need to drink at least one cup a day, and the best results have been seen when you make sure to take in the morning before starting your day.

Tea #3 A Tea for Acne

Teas have been known to help with acne as well, but you'll find that it can actually be taken internally instead of just being applied topically as well. Teas are easy to make and add into your daily routine. It is suggested to use it along with other acne remedies, as a topical and internal combination is best when you're trying to get rid of acne quickly.

Ingredients:

1. 1 Teaspoon Ginger
2. 1 Teaspoon Chamomile
3. ½ Teaspoon Spearmint

The Reason Behind It:

Acne can be caused or worsened due to inflammation, so it is best to have an herb in your tea that is meant to fight this inflammation, which is exactly why ginger was added. Chamomile also has anti-inflammation properties, but it also provides needed antioxidants to help improve the health of your skin over time. Spearmint has been added to this mix because of its antioxidant properties, helping to prevent oxidation, which helps to keep your skin from being damaged. Spearmint can act as acne prevention, making this tea a great way to reduce your likelihood of acne outbreaks.

Tea #4 A Tea for Stomach Pain

It doesn't matter what your stomach pain is from. There is no reason that you should have to deal with it, and this tea is meant to be fast acting. It has been tailored to help provide relief fast. There are a few different ingredients to make it a little more versatile as well. It's best to have it made in advance.

Ingredients:

1. ½ Teaspoon Ginger
2. 1 Teaspoon Mint

3. ½ Teaspoon Basil
4. 1 Teaspoon Licorice

The Reason Behind It:

Ginger, as most people know, is a great way to get rid of nausea quickly. It even works for morning sickness, and it stimulates your digestive system. Mint is also great at stimulating the digestive system, and it's a taste that many people can deal with, helping to make it easier to take the tea when you're feeling sickened by food. Basil is a common spice that you already have dried, but it can help because it treats muscle spasms in the abdominal region as well as limiting gas. Licorice is added to help with general indigestion and bloating.

Tea #5 A Tea for the Flu

You can also use this tea for a cold, but it's going to help cut the time you have to deal with the flu in half. Better yet, it will help to treat the symptoms that you're having to deal with immediately, making dealing with the cold or flu a little more bearable.

Ingredients:

1. ½ Teaspoon Ginger
2. 1 Teaspoon Sage
3. ½ Teaspoon Cinnamon
4. 1 Teaspoon Lemongrass

The Reason Behind It:

If you've ever dealt with the cold or flu, you already know that you're most likely to deal with stomach upset. It's best to cut it off before it happens, and drinking ginger can do that. Sage is also a common herb that you'll find dried, and it's a great source of antioxidants that will help to boost your immune system to help fight your virus. Cinnamon is added to help as a decongestant, as it's sure to help you clear your nasal passages, helping you to breathe a little better. Lemongrass is known to help with a cold or flu because it can treat both fever and cough, which are common symptoms of both the cold and flu.

Tea #6 A Tea for Fever

It doesn't matter why you have a fever, it is important that you break it. A fever isn't just uncomfortable. A fever is actually unhealthy, and it can affect your sleep and lower your immune system because of it. This tea is designed to help you break your fever quickly, and all dried herbs will work just fine.

Ingredients:

1. 2 Teaspoons Feverfew

2. 1 Teaspoon Lemongrass
3. 1 Teaspoon Peppermint
4. ½ Teaspoon White Willow

The Reason Behind It:

You are going to want to keep feverfew on hand, even though it's not a normal spice to have lying around in your cabinet. Feverfew is adeptly named, helping you to break a fever quickly. Lemongrass is also known to help you break a fever, but it was also added because it helps to flavor the tea. Peppermint will sooth your stomach and help to induce sleep, which is needed when getting over a fever. White willow will help with the pain as well as breaking the fever that caused it.

Tea #7 A Tea for Stress

It doesn't matter why you're stressed. It doesn't help your body if you're stressed for long periods of time. Make sure to handle your stress in a healthy and natural manner, and this tea will help you with that. It'll help you to lower anxiety and stave off depression. When you're stressed for long periods of time, it can lower your immune system, proving a huge detriment to your health.

Ingredients:

1. 2 Teaspoons Lavender
2. 1 Teaspoon Chamomile
3. 1 Teaspoon St. John's Wort

The Reason Behind It:

The lavender is added for its aromatherapy effects, but it is also known to relieve stress when it is taken internally. Another reason it was added to this tea is to promote the flavor. Chamomile will help you get to sleep, relaxing your muscles and treating anxiety. St. John's
18

Wort has a lot of healing benefits, but it has been added to this recipe mainly to release nervous tension.

A Little Reminder:

When you're making these teas, you should make them with precaution. Add honey and lemon if you are experiencing a sore throat. Make sure that you strain out all of the herbs before you drink the tea. You will get a better result with your tea if you boil the water on the stove, and then add the herbs while you reduce it to a simmer. Do not just turn the heat off. Then you can let it cool after straining the herbs, adding what you want to make it an acceptable drink. For flavor, peppermint can be added to almost any of these herbal recipes. Many people will also add various dried fruits, helping to flavor the tea so that they can get the medicinal benefits of these dried herbs without having to worry about sacrificing taste.

Chapter 3. Using Various Herbs in Herbal Baths

Having fresh herbs to work with is usually best, but they're not always needed, especially when hot water is added to the equation. Never dismiss the healing abilities of an herbal bath, and all of the herbs listed in the remedies below can be completely dry when you put them in the bath. You'll still find that they work just fine to help relieve you of what they're supposed to. Just remember that you need to soak for at least twenty minutes to really gain the benefits of these herbal baths. So don't rush out of the water.

Recipe #1 Herbal Bath for Stress

21

One of the most common reasons that people use an herbal bath is if they are feeling stressed, anxious, or even depressed. There are many herbs that you can use in a bath that is meant to help relieve these issues, as there are many herbs that have therapeutic properties, and almost any herbal bath will have the added benefit of helping to release stress at least a little bit. Of course, this one is directly designed to help with the issue.

Ingredients:

1. 5 Tablespoons Chamomile
2. 2 Tablespoons Lavender
3. 3 Tablespoons Lemon Balm

The Reasons Behind It:

If you're looking for a bath that is soothing, then you're almost always going to want to add chamomile. You can grow and dry chamomile easily, and it's going to promote the release of tension, even though it does not directly work on your muscles. Lavender is also something that is easy to get ahold of and dry, especially if you grow it yourself. It is known for having aromatherapy qualities to it, and you will notice this once it's been added to the water. Lemon balm is added to the list because it can help with anxiety as well as help you to sleep. This is not an herbal bath you want if you're trying to wake up in the morning.

Recipe #2 Herbal Bath for Sunburn

There are many herbs that can help with sunburn, but think of adding milk as well to the mix. It's not a dried herb, but it can help promote healing and keep your skin from getting too tight. It can even help to pull out the heat. Apple cider vinegar can also be added to this herbal bath to help you get rid of your sunburn quickly. If you do decide to add apple cider vinegar, don't add more than three to four capfuls, as it can also irritate your sunburn if you add too much of it.

Ingredients:

1. 8 Tablespoons Peppermint
2. 2 Tablespoons Meadowsweet
3. 3 Tablespoons Nettle

The Reason Behind It:

Peppermint has soothing qualities, and soaking in it is going to help take the heat out of your sunburn immediately, treating the pain that the sunburn has caused you. Meadowsweet will even help if you've already blistered from the sunburn, and it has a soothing scent that is going to help you relax as well. Nettle is added into the herbal bath because it'll help to remove the inflammation that is causing your sunburn to be worse than it would be without it.

Recipe #3 Herbal Bath for Sleep

If you're having a hard time getting to sleep, you probably already know that a warm bath helps. However, sometimes helping isn't enough. You'll be able to get to sleep better if you're using an herbal bath that is designed to help you calm yourself down and promote healthy sleep patterns. Even insomnia can be relieved by soaking in an herbal bath.

Ingredients:

1. 4 Tablespoons Passionflower
2. 2 Teaspoons Valerian
3. 2 Teaspoons Lemon Balm

The Reason Behind It:

If you're wondering why passionflower is used in a bath, it is known to help relax your muscles as it is a sedative. This can also help to promote better sleep, and it can be used to treat insomnia. Valerian is used for the same reasons, and if you don't have actual valerian around, you can use a premade valerian tea. Lemon balm was used for its anti-anxiety qualities, and it will also help for the bath to have aromatherapy qualities as well.

Recipe #4 Herbal Bath for Rejuvenation

If you're looking to wake up and feel better overall, there is an herbal bath for that. You can still use dried herbs, making it easier, and you can even make up these baths in advance. For some people some of the ingredients are a stimulant, so never soak in this bath right before you go to bed.

Ingredients:

1. 2 Teaspoons Comfrey Leaf
2. 2 Teaspoons Rosemary
3. 2 Teaspoons Nettle
4. 2 Teaspoons Rosehips

The Reason Behind It:

Comfrey leaf is known for its healing abilities, and that is because of its high vitamin C content as well as high Calcium content, which stimulates the body's natural healing abilities. Rosemary has been added to this herbal bath because it helps with any skin irritations that you may be experiencing, as well as being very fragrant and promotes the release of tension. Nettle is known to help with any inflammation you may be experiencing, and it can help clear up any skin problems you may be having. Rosehips is often used in a rejuvenating bath because of its fragrant nature, but it also has anti-aging effects due to the high antioxidant level. This can even help to clear up acne.

Recipe #5 Herbal Bath for Sore Muscles

If you're dealing with sore muscles, you're likely to be unable to really function or enjoy your day. Sore muscles can even keep you from sleeping and affect your next day. There is no reason to deal with sore muscles, and after thirty minutes in this bath, you'll find that you'll feel better immediately.

Ingredients:

1. 1 Tablespoon Sage
2. 2 Tablespoons Peppermint
3. 4 Tablespoons Lavender

The Reason Behind It:

Sage is considered to be a stimulating bath herb, and it'll help you to relax your muscles quickly. It has an earthy scent that you can enjoy, but it's great when you put it with peppermint. Peppermint is known to help relieve pain, especially the pain from sore muscles. Lavender promotes relaxation, which will help you to get the most out of this herbal soak, and it'll help you to unwind, releasing the tension that you're holding in your muscles and relaxing them during your soak.

Recipe #6 Herbal Bath for Rashes

Rashes aren't always fixed by creams, and if you want to help heal your rash in a natural way, you may find this herbal soak will help. Different rashes will react differently, but you need to try to soak at least once daily if you want your rash to go away quickly. When you're dealing with a rash, it is also great to add olive oil or oatmeal to your bath.

Ingredients:

1. 3 Tablespoons Lavender
2. 3 Tablespoons Chamomile
3. 2 Teaspoons Cinnamon
4. 1 Teaspoon Yarrow

The Reason Behind It:

Lavender isn't just a relaxing herb, but it actually has antiseptic properties as well. It is even an anti-inflammatory, helping with any inflammation that you may be experiencing as a result of your rash. Chamomile is more than just for relaxation as well, and you'll find that it promotes natural healing, helping you to heal from your rash quickly. Cinnamon is an anti-inflammatory and an antiseptic. It can help to heal fungal rashes as well, which is why it's great to add to this herbal bath. Yarrow is also a great rash treatment when added to an herbal bath, and it's great for inflammation and a variety of skin irritations.

Recipe #7 Herbal Bath for Arthritis

If you're experiencing arthritis and don't want to take a tea, then you can try an herbal bath instead, and this is a great one. Herbal baths will help your entire body if you have crippling arthritis, and all you have to do is lay there.

Ingredients:

1. 2 Teaspoons Willow Bark
2. 2 Teaspoons Cinnamon
3. 4 Teaspoons Green Tea Leaves

The Reason Behind It:

Willow bark is known for relieving pain and inflammation, which are the main problems you'll need relieved with crippling arthritis. Cinnamon is also known for helping with inflammation, and it'll help to improve any skin conditions while you're soaking in the bath. Green tea is also known for its effects on arthritis, and it is a soothing soak to use. It will even help your skin along the way.

A Little Reminder:

If you're using an herbal soak, you should notice results immediately when you get out of the bath. Soak for thirty to forty minutes, but remember that you cannot soak in cold water and expect it to have an effect on what you're trying to heal. The benefits come from the dried herbs being exposed to the hot water and then having direct and prolonged contact with your skin. There are many other ingredients besides dried herbs that you can use when you're using an herbal bath as well, so just feel free to add them in.

For example, baking soda is known to calm you down as well as relieve any irritation that you may be experiencing. Lemon juice will help to revive you as well as shrink your pores, which can help with acne as well. Salt, including Epsom salts, are known to help relax you, reduce pain, and relieve inflammation. Honey can even be used to help you hydrate your skin and for its anti-aging properties.

Chapter 4. Making Tinctures from Dried Herbs

You can make tinctures from fresh or dried herbs, and you can make them up in advance. The benefits of an herbal tincture will all depend on the herbs that you are using, but alcoholic herbal tinctures are known to work the best. That's what will be covered in this chapter. Before getting started, you need to know how to make an herbal tincture, and then recipes and there benefits can be discussed.

To make a tincture, you're going to need to have an alcohol that is consumable, and 80 proof vodka is recommended. You'll need at least a pint sized glass jar that has a screw on lid that is airtight. You will need the herbs of your choice, and then you can fill the jar halfway with the dried herbs, and then you fill the rest of it with alcohol. This is why in the coming recipes, you will not see measurements. It all depends on the size jar that you're using.

Once your herbs are in half of the jar, you are going to want to fill the rest of the jar with the alcohol. You will then need to let it sit for three weeks to six months. The longer it sits, the stronger the tincture is, and then you'll want to strain it. Most people will use a cheesecloth. The tincture can then be stored in glass jars out of the light.

A tincture boils down to being a liquid extract that you can use directly. Tinctures are taken by the dropper most of the time, and they're used at least once daily. Many people will mix them into water to take them directly if they can. You have to be careful with some tinctures.

Tincture #1 Herbal Remedy for Sleep

If you're having a hard time sleeping, then this tincture is a great help. You can make from dried herbs, and have it hanging around for whenever you need it. It's quicker to use than an herbal bath.

Ingredients:

1. 1 Part Catnip
2. 2 Parts Chamomile
3. 1 Part Lavender

The Reason Behind It:

Catnip isn't just for cats, and it is great at promoting natural sleep because it helps to fight anxiety and stress. Chamomile is known to help you relax your muscles and promote stress as well, and lavender is great with stress and inflammation, making a perfect tincture mixture for sleep.

Tincture #2 Herbal Remedy for Digestion

If you're having indigestion problems, then try out this easy to make and easy to use tincture. The best part is that it is easy to make, and all of the ingredients are easy to find.

Ingredients:

1. 2 Parts Peppermint
2. 1 Part Ginger
3. 1 Part Fennel Seeds

The Reason Behind It:

You'll find that peppermint helps you to stimulate digestive juices while relaxing your muscles, including those in your digestive track. Ginger is known to help aid with your nausea, and it's even stronger when you've made it into a tincture, helping it to worker quicker as well. Fennel seeds are also known to help with stomach pain, and it can reduce bloating.

Tincture #3 Herbal Remedy for Anxiety

If you're dealing with anxiety regularly, a tea may not be for you. You can always add a few drops of this tincture safely into your water, and drink it once daily. Of course, there are also other ways to use this tincture as well.

Ingredients:

1. 1 Part Licorice Root
2. 2 Parts Lavender

3. 1 Part Chamomile

4. 1 Part Sage

The Reason Behind It:

One of the main reasons that people will choose licorice if they are dealing with anxiety is because it can help to calm the effects that anxiety can have on the body. For example, it can help to calm your stomach and resulting nausea. It can also help to help anxiety and stress as a whole. Lavender is anti-anxiety as well, but it also will help to relieve the tension in your muscles, and this is the same reason that chamomile is added. Sage will help you to feel a little more refreshed, but it is also an anti-anxiety.

Tincture #4 Herbal Remedy for Menstrual Pain

Dealing with menstrual pain is hard, but this tincture can be taken once daily if you're using it to help you with the pain. Of course, make sure not to take more than about three to four drops, especially if it's strong.

Ingredients:

1. 1 Part Lemon Balm
2. 1 Part Stinging Nettle

The Reason Behind It:

Lemon balm is going to lower your stress levels, which will automatically help to relieve your symptoms. Of course, it will also help you relax and elevate your mood as well. One of the best parts is that it won't make you feel too drowsy, either. Of course, stinging nettle was added because it will lift your immune system, and it will help you to build up your immune system.

You'll be able to replenish the minerals and vitamins that you've lost.

Tincture #5 Herbal Remedy for Pain

This isn't a major pain reliever, but it will help you with some pain. Take it carefully, and remember to take only a few drops. Of course, you can take it once daily. Take it on the onset of pain, and do not use this tincture as a preventive measure. Due to the nature of these ingredients, you'll notice exact measurements in this tincture recipe. They can be dangerous if you use too much. You should only add a cup of 100 proof vodka to the measurements below.

Ingredients:

1. 4 Tablespoons Devil Claw
2. 2 Tablespoons Skullcap
3. 1 Teaspoon Ginger

The Reason Behind It:

Devil's Claw is known to be helpful for a lot of different types of pain, including migraines and arthritis pain. It can also help with muscle pain, so it has been added to this tincture. Skullcap promotes sleep, helps with anxiety, and is great at helping with headaches as well as migraines. Ginger is known to help your digestive system, which can add onto pain as well.

A Little Reminder:

Remember that not all herbs can be used with medical conditions, pregnancy, or allergies. If you are using a tincture, due to how strong they are, you should always ask your doctor to see if it's safe for you. You should also make them aware of how often you are going to use the tincture and exactly what went into it. If you want a tincture that is a little less strong, then you can add half vodka and half water. You can make a tincture out of a single dried herb as well. For example, you can focus on making just a lavender tincture, a chamomile one, a lemon balm one, or even a peppermint one. You can then use this later for baths, teas, or other herbal remedies, making your dried herbs change into something that is a little easier and more versatile to use. They'll even be stronger and keep longer in their tincture form due to the alcohol that you're using to make the tincture acting as a preservative.

Chapter 5. Making Powerful Salves for Healing

With dried herbs, you are also able to make a salve to help with a variety of issues. So don't worry about your herbs being dried, and you'll be able to use them either way. Of course, you need to know how to make a general salve before you can use your dried herbs to do so. There are some basic ingredients that you'll need. Make sure that you have olive oil, a double boiler, and beeswax to start with. It is best if you get your beeswax in one ounce bars, as it'll be easier to use. It's not an exact science, but it's easier to make than most tinctures, and dried herbs will never pose a problem.

Salve #1 General Healing

If you're looking to heal something like a bruise or a cut, then this is a great healing salve, and it's easy to make. So don't worry about spending too much time. Just put it in an airtight container to make sure that it doesn't go bad.

Ingredients:

1. 2 Cups Comfrey Leaves, Crushed
2. 2 Cups Olive Oil
3. ½ Cup Beeswax
4. 1 Ounce Beeswax
5. 1 Teaspoon Vitamin E
6. 2 Ounces Shea Butter

Directions:

1. Start by packing a one quart glass jar with comfrey leaves, and then fill it with

olive oil. This should infuse for at least one month. If you already have a comfrey tincture, then you can use it.

2. Use 1 ½ cups of the infused oil, and then bring it to a boil on a double boiler. Turn it down to simmer afterwards, adding the wax.

3. Melt the Shea butter into it when the other is melted.

4. Add in the vitamin E, stirring it. Pour into a container to use the salve later.

The Reason Behind It:

Comfrey is great at helping to promote natural healing for your body, and the Shea butter is going to make sure that it doesn't irritate your skin. This is a salve that you can use two to three times daily for the best results. You can even use this salve on bruises to make them heal faster.

Salve #2 A Salve for Dry Skin

Dry skin can lead to irritation and rashes, so it's best to cut it off before it even gets started, and this is an easy salve to use. It's actually considered to be a balm, and you only need four simple ingredients.

Ingredients:

1. 1 Teaspoon Cinnamon
2. 4 Tablespoons Coconut Oil
3. 1 Teaspoon Honey
4. 1 Tablespoon Beeswax

Directions:

1. All you have to do is heat everything together, combining it thoroughly. Once again, a double boiler is usually best.
2. Put it in a clean container that is airtight. It is best to use glass.

47

The Reason Behind It:

The cinnamon will help to make sure that any infection in your skin or irritation will be cleaned, while the honey and coconut oil are going to moisturize your skin. This isn't a salve that makes a lot, but you can use it as much as you like, and many people will double the recipe. Feel free to add a fragrant essential oil. Rose is a common essential oil to add.

Salve #3 A Burn Salve

It doesn't matter if you're using it for a severe or simple burn. There is no reason to wait for it to heal naturally when you can promote quicker healing with this burn salve. It's easy to make, and it's best that you have it made in advance.

Ingredients:

1. 1 Cup Almond Oil

2. 1 Ounce Comfrey Leaves
3. 1 Ounce Calendula Flowers
4. 1 Ounce Plantain Leaf
5. 1 Ounce St. John's Wort Flowers
6. 1 Ounce Beeswax
7. 40 Drops Essential Oil of Your Choice

Directions:

1. You'll want to put your dried herbs and olive oil in a double boiler, and keep the heat on low for sixty minutes. Remember to stir. This infuses the oil, and then you're going to want to strain the herbs out, removing it from heat.
2. Next, the beeswax will need to be melted in a pan. You'll do this with low heat, and then add it into the infused oil, adding in your essential oil.

3. Make sure to mix everything together, and that's your salve. Put it into a glass jar and use it as necessary.

The Reason Behind It:

You're going to want comfrey in this burn ointment because it is going to help with any and all inflammation, and it's known to speed wound healing as well. It stimulates your body to grown new skin cells, which is needed after a burn. The calendula is known to keep bacteria away as well as being an astringent. It'll help to speed the healing as well. The plantain is also necessary because of anti-inflammatory effects, but the St. John's Wort is there because it is antibacterial and it can reduce the chance that the burn will turn into a scar.

Salve #4 Herbal Remedy for Chapped Skin

It doesn't matter if it's chapped feet, elbows, lips, or any other part of your body. This is a salve that is extremely simple to make, and you can use it just as easily. You don't have to worry about overusing it, as it can't hurt you.

Ingredients:

1. ¼ Cup Lavender Flowers
2. 3 to 4 Drops Lavender Tincture
3. 2 Tablespoons Beeswax, Grated
4. ½ Cup Olive Oil

Directions:

1. Start by infusing your oil with your lavender flowers. You'll need to put it into a saucepan, adding the flowers to it. It'll need to simmer over low heat for at least fifteen to twenty minutes.

2. Then, you'll want to strain out the lavender flowers, and start melting your beeswax.

3. Put the beeswax and infused oil together, making sure to mix them together well. Then add in the tincture, folding it in.

4. Place it in an airtight glass container for later use.

The Reason Behind It:

Lavender is great for your skin, and it'll help because of its antibacterial properties. It can sooth any skin irritations that you may be experiencing, and it's an easy salve to make.

Salve #5 Herbal Remedy for Sore Muscles

There's no reason to use over the counter medication for sore muscles, and pain killers won't be needed if you use this salve on a regular basis. It'll help to loosen up your muscles and reduce your pain almost immediately.

Ingredients:

1. 2 Teaspoons St. John's Wort Flowers
2. ½ Cup Olive Oil
3. 2 Teaspoons Cayenne Pepper
4. ½ Ounce Beeswax

Directions:

1. Infuse the oil with St. John's Wort, letting it infuse for at least twenty minutes over low heat in a medium saucepan.
2. Don't forget to get out all of the herb before you use the oil.
3. Melt your beeswax, and then you can add the oil to it. Add in the cayenne

powder until it is thoroughly mixed through. Apply as necessary.

The Reason Behind It:

St. John's Wort is known to help nerve pain, but it is known to help with muscle pain as well. Many people believe that it helps with muscle pain as well. When it's combined with the cayenne pepper, a heated effect is produced. Heat is also known to help with pain, and it will help you to relieve the tension in your muscles.

Salve #6 Herbal Remedy for Cuts

If you have a cut, and you're worried about it getting infected, then try and use this salve. It promotes natural healing, and it's going to make sure that you don't' get infected so long as you continue to put it on and keep the cut relatively clean. You'll even heal up faster while using it.

Ingredients:

1. 1/3 Cup Plantain
2. ½ Ounce Beeswax
3. ½ Cup Olive Oil
4. 1 Teaspoon Cinnamon

Directions:

1. Start by infusing your oil. You can infuse both the cinnamon and plantain this time for the best effect. Make sure to heat it in the oil for about twenty minutes.
2. Strain out all of your herbs, and then you can melt your beeswax. Add the two together, and bottle it for later.

The Reason Behind It:

The plantain is going to help promote your body to heal faster, and it has antibacterial and antiseptic properties. When you infuse the oil, you'll bring it out enough that it'll be a large help in the healing process. Of course, the cinnamon is added to help make sure the cut keeps clean. If it's too much cinnamon, you may feel a small burning sensation. Just reduce the amount of cinnamon if so.

Salve #7 Herbal Remedy for Eczema

Eczema can be both painful and embarrassing, and this salve is meant to help with eczema as well as other skin issues. Just make sure you apply it at least twice daily to get the best results. You cannot over apply this salve, and it's very nourishing for your skin as a whole.

Ingredients:

1. ¼ Cup Chickweed
2. ¼ Cup Chamomile
3. ¼ Cup Peppermint

4. ¼ Cup Beeswax
5. 1 Cup Olive Oil

Directions:

1. The olive oil needs to be warmed first, and then all of the herbs can be tossed into it to start the infusion process.
2. After twenty minutes on low heat, you can strain the herbs out.
3. Make sure to now melt your beeswax, adding in the infused oil.
4. Pour into jars, and seal tightly for later use.

The Reason Behind It:

Eczema is an inflammatory skin condition, and both chamomile and chickweed is known to help as an anti-inflammatory. They're both also very good for your skin. The peppermint give as soothing sensation to the entire mix, but it also

57

has antiseptic properties and it can help to relieve mild pain.

A Little Reminder:

You don't have to make a salve as soon as you need it. Instead, you'll find it's much easier and you're more likely to use a salve if it's been made in advance. A salve will keep for a long time, and you really don't need to worry about it going bad so long as it is airtight and has not been exposed heavily to light or any moisture. Glass jars are usually best, but tin containers are also acceptable. Try to avoid plastic when you can. You'll also make the salve making process easier if you make sure to have the infused oil already made up for future use as well. A tincture can work, but an infused oil will usually work best, especially when you're working dried herbs. If you want to make the salve making process a little cheaper so it can be used on a more regular basis, then it is recommended that you buy both your containers and beeswax in bulk to save money. If you aren't growing your own herbs and drying them, you can buy the herbs in bulk as well. Make up your salves when you do, and this way the herbs won't lose their potency.

Chapter 6. A Few Herbal Drinks Using Dried Herbs

If you're looking to use an herbal drink but aren't ready to commit to a hot tea, then you'll find that these herbal drinks are great for you. You can use dried herbs, and it'll be enough to help make sure that you stay healthy. From everything from lowering your blood pressure to helping to control your diabetes, these herbal drinks can help you. It's all about finding the right one for you. Of course, you can always ice your teas as well, but these herbal drinks are known to work a little better.

Drink #1 Treating a Bladder Infection

If you are dealing with a bladder infection, then you already know how painful it can be. There's no reason to deal with it. Just take this little shot two to three times a day, and in two to three days you should feel a little better. Some of your symptoms should be taken care of or at least slightly relieved before that.

Ingredients:

1. 6 Ounces of Water, Chilled
2. 2 Tablespoons Parsley
3. 2 Ounces Cranberry Juice
4. 1 Teaspoon Ginger

Directions:

1. Just mix everything together, and then down it. Make sure that the dried parsley doesn't stick to the bottom.

The Reason Behind It:

You may be wondering why these ingredients will help you. Water is great for a bladder infection anyway, but when you add parsley into the mix it's even better. It acts a diuretic, and it speeds up the entire healing process, which is something anyone with a bladder infection is sure to be thankful for. Cranberry juice is also known to help flush out toxins. The dried ginger also comes in handy by treating any inflammation that comes with the bladder infection territory.

Drink #2 Treating High Blood Pressure

This isn't something that is going to fix itself in a day, but you'll find that herbs are a great way to lower your high blood pressure. You don't need fresh herbs for this remedy to work, but you do need to take it twice daily, and you should notice a result within one or two weeks.

Ingredients:

2. 4 Ounces Water
3. 1 Teaspoon Cinnamon
4. 1 Teaspoon Basil
5. 2 Teaspoons Honey

Directions:

1. Just mix everything together. Taking it hot is a little easier, as it'll help you get everything mixed thoroughly. The honey will help to make sure nothing sticks to

the bottom once it's completely
dissolved into the water. Down it.

The Reason Behind It:

When you're trying to lower your blood
pressure, cinnamon is a go to herb to do so. It
doesn't just lower your blood pressure, but
you'll also find that cinnamon is a common
herb that you can add into your diet if you want
to make sure that your blood sugars stay
regulated as well. The basil is also a great way
to lower your blood pressure and the
antioxidants will help as well. The honey also
has helpful antioxidants that will keep your
immune system working while you work on
lowering your blood pressure, and it makes this
shot a little easier to handle.

Drink #3 Regulating Your Blood Sugar

If you suffer from diabetes, then you already know that it's important to make sure that you regulate your blood sugar. So this drink is great, and you can just fix it in the morning and drink it throughout the day, as needed.

Ingredients:

2. 4 Ounces Water
3. ½ Teaspoon Honey
4. ½ Teaspoon Ginger
5. ½ Teaspoon Cinnamon

Directions:

1. Mix the water and honey together first, making the honey a little easier to drink down. You can always make up more to drink during the day, and some people will even make a few cups.
2. Next, once the honey is mixed in, you can then mix the ginger and cinnamon.

If you can't take it like a shot, then you can always use a spoon to get it out. If you want it to be more of a drink, just add more water.

The Reason Behind It:

Honey is known to help you regulate your blood sugar, but when you add dried ginger and cinnamon to the mix, it is even healthier for you to help control your diabetes. The ginger will help you to increase your uptake of glucose, and the cinnamon also helps to improve blood glucose.

Drink #4 A Sore Throat Shot

It doesn't matter why you have a sore throat, but you can get rid of it easily with this drink. With eight ounces of water and the dried herbs listed, your sore throat will be feeling better in no time. It always helps more if you heat up the water. You can even do this in the microwave to help.

Ingredients:

1. 8 Ounces Water
2. 1 Teaspoon Honey
3. 1 Teaspoon Lemon Juice
4. 1 Teaspoon Garlic Powder
5. ½ Teaspoon Cayenne Powder

Directions:

1. Just mix everything together. The honey will mix better if you heat up the water beforehand.
2. Then, add in everything else. You can use just dried garlic, but if it's in powdered form it'll mix into this drink a lot easier. Sip at it until it's all gone.

The Reason Behind It:

Everyone knows that honey coats and soothes a sore throat, and it even has antibacterial properties that will help you to kick whatever is causing your sore throat. Of course, lemon is also antibacterial. However, with the dried herbs, garlic is great because it will help to boost your immune system. This will help your body to naturally fight the problem causing your sore throat. It even kills bacteria. The cayenne may sound equally unpleasant, but it can help kick your sore throat to the curb as well. Cayenne is actually known to help relieve pain, giving you relief almost immediately as well as killing the harmful bacteria.

Drink #5 Cough Soothing Shot

Once again, this is best if you take it in a shot. It doesn't matter if the water is warm or cold, but the honey will mix better if it's heated up. It'll dissolve either way if you have the patience, though. Kick your cough, and use this recipe to take a shot at least three times daily.

Ingredients:

1. 4 Ounces Water
2. ½ Teaspoon Raw Honey
3. 1 Teaspoon Thyme, Ground
4. ½ Teaspoon Black Pepper

Directions:

1. Mix everything together, and down it as fast as you can. Feel free to add more honey or water as needed.

The Reason Behind It:

Honey is going to coat and sooth your throat, which in turn will help to keep you from coughing nearly as much. However, it will also promote healing. Thyme will do the same thing, and if you're going to boil your water, you can even boil the thyme in it to get the best results. Thyme will relax your muscles, helping you to keep from coughing. Black pepper also helps to eliminate the congestion that may be accompanying your cough. You can also just take a spoonful of the thyme and pepper mixed in with a teaspoon of honey for the same results.

Drink #6 A Decongestant Drink

If you are extremely congested, then you're probably looking for quick relief. You may only have dried herbs in the cabinet, but that's just fine. You can use these dried herbs to help as a decongestant, and you'll notice results almost immediately. If you're having chronic congestion issues, take it at least twice daily during the time that you're having problems.

Ingredients:

2. 4 Ounces Water
3. 1 Teaspoon Cayenne Pepper

Directions:

1. Mix it, and drink it. Yes, it's that simple.

The Reason Behind It:

If you're looking for immediate relief, something spicy is bound to help. It'll help to clear your nasal passages almost immediately. You can always add honey if you need to, but it won't be nearly as effective if you do. Try to just down it like you would a shot, and then you'll notice that your nose and eyes may run, but the congestion is gone or at least better within minutes.

Drink #7 A Drink to Cure Stomach Pain

This drink is going to help you with stomach pain and bloating immediately. You're going to find that your digestive system runs much more smoothly afterwards, making it well worth the taste. You can make it into a tea, but most people find that this remedy is a little faster.

Ingredients:

2. ½ Teaspoon Mint Extract
3. 1 Teaspoon Dried Ginger
4. 4 Ounces Cold Water

Directions:

1. Mix it together, and drink it. Make sure that none of the ginger settles to the bottom.

The Reason Behind It:

Mint is going to sooth your stomach pain, and it's going to relax the muscles of your digestive system. It's also going to promote digestive juices. Ginger is going to treat the nausea that you're feeling while getting your digestive system back on track, helping to quickly remove what could be causing your stomach pain.

A Little Reminder:

Most of these remedies can be made into a tea if you prefer, but none of the herbs that were listed have to be fresh. They can all be dried. It may take a little longer for results this way, and it won't be as strong as if you made it into a tea. However, you'll find that each of these drinks will still help you to solve your issues. Having a tincture made from the dried herbs and adding two or three drops instead of the dried herbs will help to increase the potency of these herbal remedies.

Chapter 7. A Few Reminders to Always Keep in Mind

Of course, now you know how to dry herbs and how your dried herbs can be used to help make sure that you stay healthy. Remember that dried herbs can be used from anything from your food to helping you lower your blood pressure. You can find uses for curing a bladder infection all the way to helping you with your stress levels and lack of sleep.

Remember Your Harvest:

It doesn't matter what herb you're growing, it's important that you know when to harvest your herbs. You'll also need to know how to cut them properly. There is actually a best time to cut your herbs, and that's right before your herbs flower. This is because the leaves hold the most oil right before the entire herb flowers. The oil is what allows for the aroma and flavor, and it can increase the potency of the herb.

However, remember that not all of your herbs will flower at the same time. You'll need to pay attention, as they will flower at different times during the season. If you see buds that are new or about to open, then this is a sign that it's time to collect your harvest. If they've already flowered, you can harvest and dry them as well, but don't expect the potency to be the same.

There is even a time that is best for harvesting your herbs for the best flavor, aroma, and potency. Mid-morning is usually the best time to cut them, and this is because the leaves aren't dried out by the sun yet. Early evening is okay as well, but never cut your herbs midday. These are some of the main reasons that growing, harvesting, and drying your herbs is usually best. When you buy your herbs from someone else, you never know if they were harvested properly or not.

A Tip on Cutting Your Herbs:

When you're cutting your herbs, you should be careful as well. Remember that if you are growing herbs, there are likely to be a few different bugs crawling around. This is nothing to be ashamed of, but you need to remove the bugs before you dry them and use your herbs.

A sharp knife or scissors is usually best, especially when you're cutting branches or larger stems, which you'll find mostly with mature plants. Of course, then you'll need to shake them. This will help to remove all insects, but usually shaking gently is best. At this time, you need to examine the branch. Be sure to remove all damaged or old leaves as well.

Don't Forget to Rinse Them:

You will also need to rinse your herbs as well. It is always best to use cool water. You'll want a dry towel or at least paper towels put to the side as well. You'll want to pat them dry, making sure to remove all visible water. If you don't, your herbs are more likely to mold and have to be thrown out. Lay out each leaf on the paper towel, and never put them in more than single layers. Leaves shouldn't touch, either. Let them air-dry for a little bit before hanging them if you are using that method.

Crushing Your Herbs:

Before you use any herbs in an herbal remedy or even in just food, you will most likely want to crush them for the best results. Once dried, you can usually just let yourself crumble them. Of course, for some herbs this is harder. Rosemary can be hard to crush with your hands, so it is usually best to use a mortar and pestle.

A Tip for Tinctures:

When you're making a tincture, even though it takes at least two weeks, you should shake the tincture at least once daily. This will help to infuse the tincture with the herbs that you're using, and it'll provide the best potency. You can make a tincture with one or more herbs, but make sure that you always have a dominate herb no matter what you're making it for, as this will determine what your tincture is most commonly used for.

If you have a lot of herbs, you can make a tincture out of them in advance, and this will help you to use them even when you don't' want dried herbs laying around. It is much less likely that the tincture will go bad. However, dried herbs can due to moisture or exposure to light.

A Tip for Saving Herbs:

If your herbs are about to go bad, such as they're approaching the six month mark, you are still going to want to use them up. However, you may not have something to use them in at that particular time. It's best to make a tincture, salve, or infused oil from these herbs. This way you still have something useable from the herbs that you harvested, and if you remember to do this then nothing will ever have to go to waste.

Remember:

Dried herbs can be used for most things, and they're still great for herbal remedies. You don't need to always have fresh, but while you're harvesting, if you have an excess of fresh try to use them first. This will save you time during the drying process. Dried herbs have to be stored properly, and if you're unsure if they are still good, then you need to throw the batch out. Never use herbs that are improperly labeled, too old, or have been tampered with. This can result in you getting sick. Before you use any herbal remedy, remember that it's important to tell your doctor, especially if it's going to be a daily remedy that is worked into your everyday routine.

Printed by BoD˝in Norderstedt, Germany